Vegan Meal Prep for Begin...

1

-Ingredient Affordable ,

cipes | Save Your Time ,

lifestyle | 3

dly

thy

CAMILLA KELLEY

Table of contents

Tomato Basil Pasta

Risotto with Tomato & Herbs

Tofu Shawarma Rice

Pesto Pasta

"Cheesy" Spinach Rolls

Grilled Summer Veggies

Superfood Buddha Bowl

Burrito & Cauliflower Rice Bowl

Chapter 6: Vegetables

Lemon Garlic Broccoli

Steamed Cabbage & Carrots

Collard Greens with Shiitake Mushrooms

Garlic Pea Shoots

Mashed Potato with Carrots & Corn

Sautéed Green Beans , Mushrooms & Tomatoes

Lemon Mustard Baby Veggies

Roasted Vegetables in Balsamic Sauce

Roasted Root Vegetables

Green Beans , Roasted Red Peppers & Onions

Broccoli & Cauliflower in Lemon-Dill Sauce

Vegetable Salad in Mason Jar

Chapter 7: Grain and Bean

Sweet Spicy Beans

Edamame & Aleppo Pepper

Sushi Grain Meal

Quinoa & Snap Pea Salad

Chickpea & Quinoa

Beets , Edamame & Mixed Green Salad

Black Bean & Corn Salad

Black Beans with Rice

Slow Cooked Beans

Mango with Quinoa & Black Beans

Chapter 8: Sauces and Desserts

Tomato Salsa with Marjoram

roduction

decade ago , veganism was generally regarded in a negative light.
s were considered bizarre and plant-based diets were thought to belong to the rea
conformists and tree-hugging radicals.
mes have changed.
it may seem like veganism is just one of the many healthy diets on trend , research
tes that the demand for plant-based options will continue to rise as people becom
aware of the profound effects our food choices have on our health , the environme
stainability of food sources.
're on a vegetarian diet , making the switch to the vegan diet is relatively easy.
rse , it's also possible to go from being an omnivore to being vegan. You just need
ourself so the transition will not be too drastic or difficult.
eBook , you will learn the basics of veganism.
ill also learn how meal prep can help you stick to this lifestyle in a sustainable
er.
ay , you don't have to save yourself inside the kitchen for long hours each day
ing meals. You simply have to prepare in one batch , and then reheat whenever it'
r your meal.
nient , delicious , easy and healthy—what more can you ask for?
et started!

apter 1: Vegan Made Easy

hat is Veganism?

ording to the Vegan Society , veganism refers to "a way of living that attempts to ude all forms of animal exploitation and cruelty be it for food , clothing or any othe pose."

ther words , the vegan diet is a plant-based diet and eliminates the consumption o ry , and any product that comes from animals.

le dietary veganism is restricted to the non-consumption of animal products , othe ns of veganism eliminates that use of animal products , such as silk , leather , fur , a l.

hy Vegan?

ple who decide to go vegan do so for several reasons , one of which is to stand aga lty to animals. This is because modern farming practices often mean animals live t cages and pens under generally deplorable living conditions.

ddition , many vegans are against the killing of animals for the purpose of consum meat.

ther reason why many people switch to veganism is to protest the environmental act bought about by raising livestock. Compared to the production of plant-based rnatives , animal agriculture requires the use of more resources and leaves a high on footprint.

er health is one other major factor why veganism has become more popular in re s. Vegan diets have been linked to lower body mass index and lower body weight t-based diet has also been associated with lower risk of heart disease , cancer , ar itive impairment like Alzheimer's.

nefits of Vegan Diet

anism may seem too restrictive for many , but proponents believe the benefits weigh the challenges of having to find meat-free alternatives to meals that they w to eating.

efit # 1 - Good overall health

et that eliminates animal products and animal fats improves overall health in the wing ways:

- Non-consumption of animal fats , such as trans fats and saturated fats , w raise the level of LDL or bad cholesterol in the body leads to lower risk of disease and certain cancers.
- By avoiding the consumption of animal products , vegans avoid chemicals environmental toxins that may be transferred to humans through animal
- Because the vegan diet is naturally rich in fiber and focuses on the consul of whole grains , it can help lower blood sugar levels.
- A plant-based diet that includes probiotics could also reduce arthritis pai can lessen inflammation and improve the body's ability to absorb nutrier

efit # 2 - Improved physical fitness

en a balanced diet is followed , vegans are likely to be more physically fit than the t eating counterparts

f the reasons why is because the vegan diet is often packed with nutrients that ·rt the recovery period of the muscles in between trainings. Because of their ·mption of extra nutrients and elimination of saturated fats , vegans typically have levels of endurance and enjoy more flexibility.

is also lower tendency for injuries as the diet does not contain foods that weaken ·s and bones.

it # 3 – Better weight management

·l products are higher in fats , which equates to higher calories. Because animal ·s are eliminated from the diet , vegans are likely to be better at managing their ·t. In other words , losing weight as well as keeping the weight off is easier on a pla· ·diet.

·t # 4 – Enhanced mood

·gan diet is composed of foods that are rich in nutrients , such as unsaturated fats , -3 fatty acids , complex carbohydrates , and magnesium. These nutrients are ·ary for proper brain function , including mood regulation.

·s also suggest that microbes found in the gut affect mood and consuming fiber and ·tics as well as limiting the intake of animal fats and products help ensure that the· ·h level of good bacteria in the gut.

·elines and Rules for Eating Vegan

·are no hard and fast rules for eating vegan. However , whether consciously or ·ciously , vegans often follow these guidelines in their food choices:

- **Seasonality**

·sonal fruits and vegetables aren't just cheaper , they are also more nutritious and ·cious as they are at their peak. Consuming produce that are in season also offers · ·us of being more environment friendly as these products are often found locally.

- **Going for healthy fats**

·d fats are generally found in seeds and nuts. These fats are considered healthy ·ause they help in the absorption of other nutrients , as well as in aiding hormone ·duction and formation of cell membranes. Healthy fats also help regulate genetic ·tion.

- **Boosting protein intake**

· body needs protein to create and repair tissues and produce hormones and ·ymes. Protein also makes up the blood , skin , muscles , cartilage , and bones , whi· ·hy it is important for any diet to contain enough protein to keep a person in good ·th. The most common plant-based sources of protein are beans , legumes , nuts , ·ulina , and soy products , such as tofu , edamame , and tempeh , which are major ·ponents of most vegan diets.

- **Loading up on fiber**

· pared to their meat-eating counterparts , vegans consume more whole grains , n· ·ds , legumes , as well as vegetables and fruits. Thus , they get a fair share of fiber · · their diet.

- **Supplementing**

·ite eating a balanced diet , nutrient deficiency is common among vegans. Vitami· for example , is usually lacking in the vegan diet because it is mostly found in animal sources like beef , organ meats , sardines , clams , tuna , and trout. For this reason , vegans are advised to take vitamin B12 supplements or consume more for foods.

hat to Eat

ay , there are plenty of vegan ingredient alternatives that it's not too difficult to wh e of the meal's vegans were used to eating before going on a completely plant-bas

rt from fruits and vegetables , a typical vegan diet consists of:

- Tofu
- Tempeh
- Seitan
- Beans
- Lentils
- Seeds
- Nuts and nut milks
- Molasses and maple/rice syrup
- Ready-made vegan products like vegan meat , vegan cheese , plant-based , and others

hat Not to Eat

foods that originate from animals or contain animal products are on the do-not-ea h as:

- Beef
- Pork
- Chicken
- Fish
- Seafood
- Dairy
- Eggs
- Honey
- Foods that contain ingredients of animal origin , such as some wine and b and certain chewing gums

ps for Success

ou're already following a vegetarian diet , making the switch to an exclusively pla ed diet is much easier and has a higher chance of success. Thus , if animal produc t of most of your meals , try going vegetarian first.

can then gradually replace eggs , dairy , and fish with vegan alternatives so the s be more manageable and sustainable.

following are examples of other tips to help you successfully follow the vegan di

- Stock up on vegan staples , such as tofu , nuts , seeds , and vegan condim
- Apart from eating a balanced meal , make sure that you are getting enou the vital nutrients by taking supplements or consuming fortified foods.

- Find a group of like-minded individuals who can offer support and meal prep ideas. If you can't find vegans in your circle of friends , try checking online for social media groups or meetups that you can join.
- Many restaurants cater to people with various dietary requirements so eating out shouldn't be too difficult. However , you can always call ahead or check the establishment's website to make sure they have vegan options.
- To maximize the health benefits , you get from having a plant-based diet , it's necessary that you make the necessary lifestyle changes , such as exercising , getting adequate sleep , and managing stress.
- It's important to talk to your doctor if you have a health condition that may become aggravated by a sudden change in diet.
- Make meal planning and meal prep part of your routine.

nefits of Meal Prepping

ether you are on a vegan diet or just want to get a head start on food prep for the w
e are many reasons why meal prepping should be part of your routine. No matter
son , meal prep helps you:

efit # 1 - Save time

of the biggest benefits of meal prepping is that you save time shopping and cookir
l during the week. While some meals don't take hours to cook , it can seem too mu
ecially at the end of a very long day. When you know you have a meal ready to hea
/or eat , it relieves some of the stress and frees up time that you can use for somet
.

efit # 2 - Save money

ing food in bulk is a good way to save on grocery costs. Meal prepping also helps y
id eating out too much , especially when you have no time to shop or cook food du
week.

efit # 3 - Save energy

king a big batch of food at once uses up significantly less energy than cooking mea
ry single day.

efit # 4 - Reduce waste

d waste is a huge problem in today's society , but one way to reduce the wastage c
rough meal prepping. When you plan your meals , you'll know how much food yo
d to cook and , therefore , you'll buy only the ingredients you need. Thus , you wor
e stocks of food items that don't get used past their best before date. Moreover , b
buy food in bulk , you reduce the amount of food packaging that gets thrown awa

efit # 5 - Have control

l prepping gives you better control about what to eat and how much to eat , whic
ful if you are on a weight loss plan. For vegans , meal prep is important because y
trol the components of your meals and it helps ensure that you get enough of all t
ients your body needs.

efit # 6 - Reduce your carbon footprint

ing to and from the grocery and going to restaurants entail carbon emissions tha
reduce by shopping only once or twice a week.

e Common Mistakes by Meal Prepping Beginners

u're new to meal prepping , the following are examples of common mistakes tha
avoid:

take # 1 - Choosing the wrong recipes

e meals are best eaten immediately so it's best to avoid these when doing your r
. Meals that can be fully or partially prepared in advance , easily reheated or tha
caled up or down are excellent meal prepping recipes.

take # 2 – Not having a strategy

l prepping can seem intimidating because it requires careful planning for efficie
me and energy. However , once you get the hang of it meal prepping becomes m
ral.

thing to remember no matter what kind of meal you are making is to take note of t
1 of the cooking time as well as the steps involved in the recipe.

with the recipe that takes the longest to cook , look for opportunities for multitask
be organized in the use of kitchen appliance to minimize cleanup in between uses.

ke # 3 – Not setting aside enough time

neal prepping helps you save time but it's not something done magically. Obviously
takes time. If you don't set aside enough time for the food prep , cooking , and stor
end up so frustrated and overwhelmed you may never want to try doing it again.

arters , block off just an hour of the day to prep one or two recipes for the coming

Then , gradually increase the time and the number of recipes to work on as you

1e more confident with the process.

1

akfast: Avocado Pancakes

ch: Tomato Basil Pasta

ner: Tofu Shawarma Rice

2

akfast: Pumpkin Oats

ch: Green Beans , Roasted Red Peppers and Onions

ner: Risotto with Tomato and Herbs

3

akfast: Eggless Omelet

ch: Broccoli and Cauliflower in Lemon-Dill Sauce

ner: Vegetable Salad in Mason Jar

4

akfast: Melon Muesli

ch: "Cheesy" Spinach Rolls

ner: Pesto Pasta

5

akfast: Peanut Butter Toast with Apple Slices

ch: Vegan Tacos

ner: Edamame and Aleppo Pepper

6

akfast: Oatmeal with Pears

ch: Grilled Broccoli with Chili Garlic Oil

ner: Steamed Cabbage and Carrots

7

akfast: Hawaiian Toast

ch: Sushi Grain Meal

ner: Roasted Root Vegetables

8

akfast: Thai Oatmeal

ch: Grilled Summer Veggies

ner: Quinoa and Snap Pea Salad

9

akfast: Avocado and White Bean Toast

ch: Spinach with Walnuts & Avocado

ner: Lemon Garlic Broccoli

10

akfast: Vegan Oatmeal Waffle

ch: Sweet Spicy Beans

ner: Mashed Potato with Carrots & Corn

11

akfast: Tropical Oats

ch: Garlic Pea Shoots

r: Roasted Vegetables in Balsamic Sauce

2

fast: Toast with Refried Beans
: Sauteed Green Beans , Mushrooms and Tomatoes
r: Carrot and Radish Slaw with Sesame Dressing

3

fast: Tofu Omelet
: Grilled Barbecue Tofu
r: Chickpea and Quinoa

4

ast: Vegan Banana Bread
: Roasted Vegetables in Balsamic Sauce
: Grilled Broccoli with Chili Garlic Oil

5

ast: Sweet Potato Hash Browns
   Lemon Mustard Baby Veggies
: Sauteed Green Beans , Mushrooms and Tomatoes

6

ast: Green Smoothie
   Beets , Edamame and Mixed Green Salad
: Roasted Veggies in Lemon Sauce

7

ast: Tomato , Mushroom and Spinach Quiche
   Collard Greens with Shiitake Mushrooms
: Vegan Tacos

8

ist: Apple , Pecans and Cinnamon Oatmeal
   Broccoli & Cauliflower in Lemon-Dill Sauce
   Superfood Buddha Bowl

st: Vegan Breakfast Sandwich
Black Bean and Corn Salad
   Burrito and Cauliflower Rice Bowl

st: Cinnamon Quinoa
Mashed Potato with Carrots and Corn
   Lemon Mustard Baby Veggies

st: Pancakes with Strawberries
Spicy Snow Pea and Tofu Stir Fry
   Veggie Kebabs

st: Thai Oatmeal
Black Beans with Rice

23
akfast: Peanut Butter Toast with Apple Slices
ich: Roasted Veggies in Lemon Sauce
ner: Spinach with Walnuts and Avocado
24
akfast: Vegan French Toast
ich: Lemon Garlic Broccoli
ner: Veggie Kebabs
25
akfast: Pumpkin Oats
ich: Burrito and Cauliflower Rice Bowl
ner: Mango with Quinoa and Black Beans
26
akfast: Avocado Pancakes
ich: Carrot and Radish Slaw with Sesame Dressing
ner: Steamed Cabbage and Carrots
27
akfast: Vegan Breakfast Taco
ich: Spicy Snow Pea and Tofu Stir Fry
ner: Superfood Buddha Bowl
28
akfast: Granola Parfait
ich: Garlic Pea Shoots
ner: Grilled Summer Veggies
29
akfast: Tapioca Porridge
ich: Tofu Shawarma Rice
ner: Risotto with Tomato & Herbs
30
akfast: Banana and Nut Oatmeal
ich: Collard Greens with Shiitake Mushrooms
ner: Pesto Pasta

nut Butter Toast with Apple Slices

ration Time: 5 minutes

ng Time: 0 minute

ıg: 1

dients:

- 1 slice whole-wheat bread , toasted
- 2 tablespoons peanut butter
- ¼ cup apple , sliced
- ¼ teaspoon ground cardamom

ɔd:

1. Spread bread slice with peanut butter.
2. Top with apple slices and sprinkle with cardamom.
3. Store in a food container.

ional Value:

- *Calories 293*
- *Total Fat 17 g*
- *Saturated Fat 3 g*
- *Cholesterol 0 mg*
- *Sodium 204 mg*
- *Total Carbohydrate 21 g*
- *Dietary Fiber 5 g*
- *Total Sugars 5 g*
- *Protein 11 g*
- *Potassium 90 mg*

ocado Pancakes

paration Time: 15 minutes
king Time: 10 minutes
vings: 4
redients:

- 2 tablespoons flaxseed meal
- 5 tablespoons water
- 1 cup almond milk (unsweetened)
- 2 tablespoons sugar
- 1 cup mashed ripe avocado
- 1 teaspoon vanilla extract
- ¼ teaspoon salt
- 1 teaspoon lemon zest
- 1 ½ teaspoons baking powder
- 1 cup all-purpose flour
- 1 teaspoon oil
- Blueberries

hod:

1. Put flaxseed meal in a bowl.
2. Stir in water.
3. Let sit for 5 minutes.
4. Add milk , sugar , avocado , vanilla extract , salt and lemon zest in a blende
5. Blend until smooth.
6. Transfer mixture to a bowl and add the flaxseed mixture.
7. Stir in baking powder and flour.
8. In a pan over medium heat , add the oil.
9. Pour a small amount of the batter.
10. Flip once the surface starts to bubble.
11. Cook for 4 minutes per side.
12. Place in a food container and top with blueberries.

ritional Value:

- *Calories 258*
- *Total Fat 7 g*
- *Saturated Fat 1 g*
- *Cholesterol 0 mg*
- *Sodium 374 mg*
- *Total Carbohydrate 43 g*
- *Dietary Fiber 8 g*
- *Total Sugars 7 g*
- *Protein 5 g*
- *Potassium 370 mg*

meal with Pears

ration Time: 5 minutes

ng Time: 5 minutes

ng: 1

dients:

- ¼ cup rolled oats , cooked
- ¼ teaspoon ground ginger
- ¼ teaspoon ground cinnamon
- ¼ cup pear , sliced

od:

1. Transfer cooked oats in a glass jar with lid.
2. Stir in the ginger and cinnamon.
3. Top with pear slices.

ional Value:

- *Calories 108*
- *Total Fat 2 g*
- *Saturated Fat 0 g*
- *Cholesterol 0 mg*
- *Sodium 5 mg*
- *Total Carbohydrate 21 g*
- *Dietary Fiber 3 g*
- *Total Sugars 4 g*
- *Protein 3 g*
- *Potassium 440 mg*

ai Oatmeal

Preparation Time: 10 minutes
Cooking Time: 5 minutes
Serving: 1
Ingredients:

- ½ cup rolled oats , cooked
- 1 tablespoon peanut butter
- ½ cup coconut milk (unsweetened)
- ½ teaspoon curry powder
- 1 teaspoon tamari
- 2 tablespoons tomatoes , chopped
- ¼ cup spinach , cooked and chopped
- 1 tablespoon cilantro , chopped

Method:

1. Place oats , peanut butter , milk , curry powder and tamari in a jar.
2. Mix well.
3. Refrigerate overnight.
4. Top with tomatoes , spinach and cilantro before serving.

Nutritional Value:

- *Calories 307*
- *Total Fat 14 g*
- *Saturated Fat 4 g*
- *Cholesterol 0 mg*
- *Sodium 467 mg*
- *Total Carbohydrate 34 g*
- *Dietary Fiber 6 g*
- *Total Sugars 3 g*
- *Protein 10 g*
- *Potassium 294 mg*

pical Oats

ration Time: 10 minutes

ng Time: 5 minutes

g: 1

dients:

- ½ cup rolled oats , cooked
- ¾ cup coconut milk (unsweetened)
- 1 tablespoon dried mango , chopped
- ¼ cup pineapple , diced
- 1 ½ teaspoons chia seeds
- 1 ½ teaspoons shredded coconut (unsweetened)

d:

1. Add layers of oats , coconut milk , mango , pineapple and chia seeds in a glass with lid.
2. Seal the jar and refrigerate until ready to eat.
3. Top with the coconut shreds before serving.

ional Value:

- *Calories 281*
- *Total Fat 10 g*
- *Saturated Fat 5 g*
- *Cholesterol 0 mg*
- *Sodium 147 mg*
- *Total Carbohydrate 42 g*
- *Dietary Fiber 8 g*
- *Total Sugars 10 g*
- *Protein 7 g*
- *Potassium 205 mg*

weet Potato Hash Browns

paration Time: 10 minutes

king Time: 6 minutes

vings: 6

redients:

- 1 clove garlic , grated
- ¼ cup shallot , chopped
- 5 cups sweet potato , shredded
- 3 tablespoons olive oil , divided
- Salt and pepper to taste

thod:

1. Put the garlic , shallot , sweet potato , 1 tablespoon olive oil , salt and pepp bowl.
2. Add 1 tablespoon oil in a pan over medium heat.
3. Pour a half cup of the sweet potato patty in the pan. Flatten using a spatul:
4. Cook the patty for 3 minutes per side.
5. Cook remaining patties with the remaining oil.

ritional Value:

- *Calories 103*
- *Total Fat 7 g*
- *Saturated Fat 1 g*
- *Cholesterol 0 mg*
- *Sodium 208 mg*
- *Total Carbohydrate 9 g*
- *Dietary Fiber 1 g*
- *Total Sugars 3 g*
- *Protein 1 g*
- *Potassium 207 mg*

le , Pecans & Cinnamon Oatmeal

ıration Time: 5 minutes

ng Time: 10 minutes

ıg: 1

dients:

- ½ cup rolled oats , cooked
- ½ tablespoon chia seeds
- 1 teaspoon maple syrup
- ¼ teaspoon ground cinnamon
- ½ cup (unsweetened) almond milk
- Salt to taste
- ½ cup apple , diced
- 2 tablespoons pecans , toasted

od:

1. Layer the oats , maple syrup , cinnamon and almond milk in a glass jar.
2. Season with a little bit of salt.
3. Cover the jar and refrigerate.
4. Top with apples and pecans before serving.

ional Value:

- *Calories 215*
- *Total Fat 4 g*
- *Saturated Fat 1 g*
- *Cholesterol 0 mg*
- *Sodium 232 mg*
- *Total Carbohydrate 41 g*
- *Dietary Fiber 6 g*
- *Total Sugars 11 g*
- *Protein 6 g*
- *Potassium 249 mg*

mpkin Oats

paration Time: 5 minutes
king Time: 0 minute
ving: 1

redients:

- ½ cup rolled oats , cooked
- ½ cup soy milk
- 2 teaspoons maple syrup
- 3 tablespoons pumpkin puree
- ½ teaspoon vanilla extract
- ¼ teaspoon ground cinnamon
- Salt to taste
- Toasted pumpkin seeds

hod:

1. Mix the oats , soy milk , maple syrup , pumpkin puree , vanilla extract and cinnamon in a glass jar with lid.
2. Season with a pinch of salt.
3. Seal the jar and refrigerate.
4. Top with pumpkin seeds before serving.

ritional Value:

- *Calories 182*
- *Total Fat 4 g*
- *Saturated Fat 1 g*
- *Cholesterol 0 mg*
- *Sodium 351 mg*
- *Total Carbohydrate 41 g*
- *Dietary Fiber 6 g*
- *Total Sugars 11 g*
- *Protein 6 g*
- *Potassium 290 mg*

vaiian Toast

Preparation Time: 5 minutes

ng Time: 5 minutes

ng: 1

dients:

- 1 slice whole wheat bread , toasted
- 3 teaspoons tomato sauce
- 1 pineapple ring
- 3 teaspoons vegan cheese , shredded

od:

1. Spread tomato sauce on the toast.
2. Pu the pineapple ring on top.
3. Top with shredded cheese.
4. Bake in the oven until the cheese has melted.
5. Store in a food container
6. Reheat before serving.

ional Value:

- *Calories 252*
- *Total Fat 11 g*
- *Saturated Fat 2 g*
- *Cholesterol 0 mg*
- *Sodium 230 mg*
- *Total Carbohydrate 33 g*
- *Dietary Fiber 5 g*
- *Total Sugars 8 g*
- *Protein 8 g*
- *Potassium 54 mg*

gless Omelette

paration Time: 10 minutes

king Time: 5 minutes

vings: 2

redients:

- 1 tablespoon olive oil
- 1 onion , sliced into strips
- 1 red bell pepper , sliced into strips
- 1 tomato , sliced into strips
- 4 servings vegan egg , beaten

hod:

1. Pour the oil in a pan over medium heat.
2. Add the onion , red bell pepper and tomato and cook for 2 to 3 minutes.
3. Transfer vegetables to a bowl.
4. Add the vegan eggs to the bowl.
5. Pour the mixture to the pan.
6. Cook for 3 minutes or until firm.
7. Store in a food container.
8. Reheat before serving.

ritional Value:

- *Calories 107*
- *Total Fat 7.3g*
- *Saturated Fat 1g*
- *Cholesterol 0mg*
- *Sodium 5mg*
- *Total Carbohydrate 10.9g*
- *Dietary Fiber 2.4g*
- *Total Sugars 6.2g*
- *Protein 1.5g*
- *Potassium 266mg*

on Muesli

ration Time: 10 minutes

ng Time: 5 minutes

gs: 2

dients:

- ½ cup muesli cereal (uncooked)
- ½ cup almond milk (unsweetened)
- ½ cup water
- ½ cup fresh cantaloupe , chopped
- 1 pinch ground cinnamon

d:

1. In a heat proof bowl , mix the cereal , milk and water.
2. Microwave in high power for 5 minutes.
3. Top with the cantaloupe and season with cinnamon before serving.

ional Value:

- *Calories 96*
- *Total Fat 2 g*
- *Saturated Fat 0 g*
- *Cholesterol 0 mg*
- *Sodium 102 mg*
- *Total Carbohydrate 20 g*
- *Dietary Fiber 2 g*
- *Total Sugars 10 g*
- *Protein 3 g*
- *Potassium 259 mg*

ocado & White Bean Toast

paration Time: 5 minutes

king Time: 0 minute

ving: 1

redients:

- ¼ avocado , mashed
- 1 slice whole-wheat bread , toasted
- ½ cup canned white beans , rinsed and drained
- Salt and pepper to taste

thod:

1. Spread mashed avocado on toasted bread.
2. Top with white beans.
3. Season with salt and pepper.

ritional Value:

- *Calories 230*
- *Total Fat 9 g*
- *Saturated Fat 1 g*
- *Cholesterol 0 mg*
- *Sodium 459 mg*
- *Total Carbohydrate 35 g*
- *Dietary Fiber 11 g*
- *Total Sugars 3 g*
- *Protein 11 g*
- *Potassium 655 mg*

gie & Tofu Kebabs

ration Time: 15 minutes

ng Time: 12 minutes

gs: 4

dients:

- 2 cloves garlic , minced
- ¼ cup balsamic vinegar
- ¼ cup olive oil
- 1 tablespoon Italian seasoning
- Salt and pepper to taste
- 1 onion , sliced into quarters
- 12 medium mushrooms
- 16 cherry tomatoes
- 1 zucchini , sliced into rounds
- 1 cup tofu , cubed
- 4 cups cauliflower rice

d:

1. In a bowl , mix the garlic , vinegar , oil , Italian seasoning , salt and pepper.
2. Toss the vegetable slices and tofu in the mixture.
3. Marinate for 1 hour.
4. Thread into 8 skewers and grill for 12 minutes , turning once or twice.
5. Add cauliflower rice into 4 food containers.
6. Add 2 kebab skewers on top of each container of cauliflower rice.
7. Reheat kebabs in the grill before serving.

ional Value:

- *Calories 58*
- *Total Fat 2 g*
- *Saturated Fat 0 g*
- *Cholesterol 0 mg*
- *Sodium 84 mg*
- *Total Carbohydrate 9 g*
- *Dietary Fiber 2 g*
- *Total Sugars 5 g*
- *Protein 2 g*
- *Potassium 509 mg*

rrot and Radish Slaw with Sesame Dressing

paration Time: 10 minutes

king Time: 0 minute

vings: 4

redients:

- 2 tablespoons sesame oil , toasted
- 3 tablespoons rice vinegar
- ½ teaspoon sugar
- 2 tablespoons low sodium tamari
- 1 cup carrots , sliced into strips
- 2 cups radishes , sliced
- 2 tablespoons fresh cilantro , chopped
- 2 teaspoons sesame seeds , toasted

hod:

1. Mix the oil , vinegar , sugar and tamari in a bowl.
2. Add the carrots , radishes and cilantro.
3. Toss to coat evenly.
4. Let sit for 10 minutes.
5. Transfer to a food container.

ritional Value:

- *Calories 98*
- *Total Fat 8 g*
- *Saturated Fat 1 g*
- *Cholesterol 0 mg*
- *Sodium 336 mg*
- *Total Carbohydrate 6 g*
- *Dietary Fiber 2 g*
- *Total Sugars 3 g*
- *Protein 2 g*
- *Potassium 241 mg*

cy Snow Pea and Tofu Stir Fry

ration Time: 20 minutes

ng Time: 20 minutes

ags: 4

dients:

- 1 cup unsalted natural peanut butter
- 2 teaspoons brown sugar
- 2 tablespoons reduced-sodium soy sauce
- 2 teaspoons hot sauce
- 3 tablespoons rice vinegar
- 14 oz. tofu
- 4 teaspoons oil
- 1/4 cup onion , sliced
- 2 tablespoons ginger , grated
- 3 cloves garlic , minced
- 1/2 cup broccoli , sliced into florets
- 1/2 cup carrot , sliced into sticks
- 2 cups fresh snow peas , trimmed
- 2 tablespoons water
- 2 cups brown rice , cooked
- 4 tablespoons roasted peanuts (unsalted)

d:

1. In a bowl , mix the peanut butter , sugar , soy sauce , hot sauce and rice vineg
2. Blend until smooth and set aside.
3. Drain the tofu and sliced into cubes.
4. Pat dry with paper towel.
5. Add oil to a pan over medium heat.
6. Add the tofu and cook for 2 minutes or until brown on all sides.
7. Transfer the tofu to a plate.
8. Add the onion , ginger and garlic to the pan.
9. Cook for 2 minutes.
10. Add the broccoli and carrot.
11. Cook for 5 minutes.
12. Stir in the snow peas.
13. Pour in the water and cover.
14. Cook for 4 minutes.
15. Add the peanut sauce to the pan along with the tofu.
16. Heat through for 30 seconds.
17. In a food container , add the brown rice and top with the tofu and vegetable fry.
18. Top with roasted peanuts.

nal Value:

- *Calories 514*
- *Total Fat 27 g*

- *Saturated Fat 4 g*
- *Cholesterol 0 mg*
- *Sodium 376 mg*
- *Total Carbohydrate 49 g*
- *Dietary Fiber 7 g*
- *Total Sugars 12 g*
- *Protein 22 g*
- *Potassium 319 mg*

sted Veggies in Lemon Sauce

ration Time: 15 minutes

ng Time: 20 minutes

gs: 5

dients:

- 2 cloves garlic , sliced
- 1 ½ cups broccoli florets
- 1 ½ cups cauliflower florets
- 1 tablespoon olive oil
- Salt to taste
- 1 teaspoon dried oregano , crushed
- ¾ cup zucchini , diced
- ¾ cup red bell pepper , diced
- 2 teaspoons lemon zest

d:

1. Preheat your oven to 425 degrees F.
2. In a baking pan , add the garlic , broccoli and cauliflower.
3. Toss in oil and season with salt and oregano.
4. Roast in the oven for 10 minutes.
5. Add the zucchini and bell pepper to the pan.
6. Stir well.
7. Roast for another 10 minutes.
8. Sprinkle lemon zest on top before serving.
9. Transfer to a food container and reheat before serving.

onal Value:

- *Calories 52*
- *Total Fat 3 g*
- *Saturated Fat 0 g*
- *Cholesterol 0 mg*
- *Sodium 134 mg*
- *Total Carbohydrate 5 g*
- *Dietary Fiber 2 g*
- *Total Sugars 2 g*
- *Protein 2 g*
- *Potassium 270 mg*

inach with Walnuts & Avocado

paration Time: 5 minutes

king Time: 0 minute

vings: 1

redients:

- 3 cups baby spinach
- ½ cup strawberries , sliced
- 1 tablespoon white onion , chopped
- 2 tablespoons vinaigrette
- ¼ medium avocado , diced
- 2 tablespoons walnut , toasted

thod:

1. Put the spinach , strawberries and onion in a glass jar with lid.
2. Drizzle dressing on top.
3. Top with avocado and walnuts.
4. Seal the lid and refrigerate until ready to serve.
5.
6. 296 calories; 18 g fat(2 g sat); 10 g fiber; 27 g carbohydrates; 8 g protein;
7. 63 mcg folate; 0 mg cholesterol; 11 g sugars; 0 g added sugars; 11 ,084 IU vitamin A; 103 mg
8. vitamin C; 192 mg calcium; 7 mg iron; 195 mg sodium; 385 mg

tritional Value:

- *Calories 296*
- *Total Fat 18 g*
- *Saturated Fat 2 g*
- *Cholesterol 0 mg*
- *Sodium 195 mg*
- *Total Carbohydrate 27 g*
- *Dietary Fiber 10 g*
- *Total Sugars 11 g*
- *Protein 8 g*
- *Potassium 103 mg*

an Tacos

ration Time: 20 minutes
ng Time: 10 minutes
gs: 4

dients:

- ½ teaspoon onion powder
- ½ teaspoon garlic powder
- 1 teaspoon chili powder
- 2 tablespoons tamari
- 16 oz. tofu , drained and crumbled
- 1 tablespoon olive oil
- 1 ripe avocado
- 1 tablespoon vegan mayonnaise
- 1 teaspoon lime juice
- Salt to taste
- 8 corn tortillas , warmed
- ½ cup fresh salsa
- 2 cups iceberg lettuce , shredded
- Pickled radishes

d:

1. Combine the onion powder , garlic powder , chili powder and tamari in a bow
2. Marinate the tofu in the mixture for 10 minutes.
3. Pour the oil in a pan over medium heat.
4. Cook the tofu mixture for 10 minutes.
5. In another bowl , mash the avocado and mix with mayo , lime juice and salt.
6. Stuff each corn tortilla with tofu mixture , mashed avocado , salsa and lettuce
7. Serve with pickled radishes.

ional Value:

- *Calories 360*
- *Total Fat 21 g*
- *Saturated Fat 3 g*
- *Cholesterol 0 mg*
- *Sodium 610 mg*
- *Total Carbohydrate 33 g*
- *Dietary Fiber 8 g*
- *Total Sugars 4 g*
- *Protein 17 g*
- *Potassium 553 mg*

illed Broccoli with Chili Garlic Oil

paration Time: 15 minutes

king Time: 16 minutes

vings: 4

redients:

- 3 tablespoons olive oil , divided
- 2 tablespoons vegetable broth (unsalted)
- 2 cloves garlic , sliced thinly
- 1 chili pepper , julienned
- 1 1/2 lb. broccoli , sliced into florets
- Salt and pepper to taste
- 2 lemons , sliced in half

hod:

1. Preheat your grill to medium-high.
2. In a bowl , mix 1 tablespoon oil , garlic , broth and chili.
3. Heat in a pan over medium heat for 30 seconds.
4. In another bowl , toss the broccoli florets in salt , pepper and remaining o
5. Grill the broccoli florets for 10 minutes.
6. Grill the lemon slices for 5 minutes.
7. Toss the grilled broccoli and lemon in chili garlic oil.
8. Store in a food container and reheat before serving.

ritional Value:

- *Calories 164*
- *Total Fat 11 g*
- *Saturated Fat 1 g*
- *Cholesterol 0 mg*
- *Sodium 208 mg*
- *Total Carbohydrate 12 g*
- *Dietary Fiber 2 g*
- *Total Sugars 4 g*
- *Protein 6 g*
- *Potassium 519 mg*

nato Basil Pasta

ration Time: 5 minutes

ng Time: 10 minutes

gs: 4

dients:

- 2 cups low-sodium vegetable broth
- 2 cups water
- 8 oz. pasta
- 1 ½ teaspoons Italian seasoning
- 15 oz. canned diced tomatoes
- 2 tablespoons olive oil
- ½ teaspoon garlic powder
- ½ teaspoon onion powder
- ¼ teaspoon crushed red pepper
- ½ teaspoon salt
- 6 cups baby spinach
- ½ cup basil , chopped

d:

1. Add all the ingredients except spinach and basil in a pot over high heat.
2. Mix well.
3. Cover the pot and bring to a boil.
4. Reduce the heat.
5. Simmer for 5 minutes.
6. Add the spinach and cook for 5 more minutes.
7. Stir in basil.
8. Transfer to a food container.
9. Microwave before serving.

onal Value:

- *Calories 339*
- *Total Fat 10 g*
- *Saturated Fat 1 g*
- *Cholesterol 0 mg*
- *Sodium 465 mg*
- *Total Carbohydrate 55 g*
- *Dietary Fiber 8 g*
- *Total Sugars 6 g*
- *Protein 11 g*
- *Potassium 308 mg*

sotto with Tomato & Herbs

Preparation Time: 10 minutes

Cooking Time: 20 minutes

Servings: 32

Ingredients:

- 2 oz. Arborio rice
- 1 teaspoon dried garlic , minced
- 3 tablespoons dried onion , minced
- 1 tablespoon dried Italian seasoning , crushed
- ¾ cup snipped dried tomatoes
- 1 ½ cups reduced-sodium chicken broth

Method:

1. Make the dry risotto mix by combining all the ingredients except broth in a large bowl.
2. Divide the mixture into eight resealable plastic bags. Seal the bag.
3. Store at room temperature for up to 3 months.
4. When ready to serve , pour the broth in a pot.
5. Add the contents of 1 plastic bag of dry risotto mix.
6. Bring to a boil and then reduce heat.
7. Cover the pot and simmer for 20 minutes.
8. Serve with vegetables.

Nutritional Value:

- *Calories 80*
- *Total Fat 0 g*
- *Saturated Fat 0 g*
- *Cholesterol 0 mg*
- *Sodium 276 mg*
- *Total Carbohydrate 17 g*
- *Dietary Fiber 2 g*
- *Total Sugars 0 g*
- *Protein 3 g*
- *Potassium 320 mg*

Shawarma Rice

Preparation Time: 15 minutes

Cooking Time: 15 minutes

Servings: 4

Ingredients:

- 4 cups cooked brown rice
- 4 cups cooked tofu , sliced into small cubes
- 4 cups cucumber , cubed
- 4 cups tomatoes , cubed
- 4 cups white onion , cubed
- 2 cups cabbage , shredded
- 1/2 cup vegan mayo
- 1/8 cup garlic , minced
- Garlic salt to taste
- Hot sauce

Method:

1. Add brown rice into 4 food containers.
2. Arrange tofu , cucumber , tomatoes , white onion and cabbage on top.
3. In a bowl , mix the mayo , garlic , and garlic salt.
4. Drizzle top with garlic sauce and hot sauce before serving.

Nutritional Value:

- *Calories 667*
- *Total Fat 12.6g*
- *Saturated Fat 2.2g*
- *Cholesterol 0mg*
- *Sodium 95mg*
- *Total Carbohydrate 116.5g*
- *Dietary Fiber 9.9g*
- *Total Sugars 9.4g*
- *Protein 26.1g*
- *Potassium 1138mg*

sto Pasta

paration Time: 10 minutes
king Time: 8 minutes
vings: 2
redients:

- 1 cup fresh basil leaves
- 4 cloves garlic
- 2 tablespoons walnut
- 2 tablespoons olive oil
- 1 tablespoon vegan Parmesan cheese
- 2 cups cooked penne pasta
- 2 tablespoons black olives , sliced

thod:

1. Put the basil leaves , garlic , walnut , olive oil and Parmesan cheese in a foo processor.
2. Pulse until smooth.
3. Divide pasta into 2 food containers.
4. Spread the basil sauce on top.
5. Top with black olives.
6. Store until ready to serve.

ritional Value:

- *Calories 374*
- *Total Fat 21.1g*
- *Saturated Fat 2.6g*
- *Cholesterol 47mg*
- *Sodium 92mg*
- *Total Carbohydrate 38.6g*
- *Dietary Fiber 1.1g*
- *Total Sugars 0.2g*
- *Protein 10g*
- *Potassium 215mg*

eesy" Spinach Rolls

ration Time: 20 minutes
ng Time: 15 minutes
1gs: 6

dients:

- 18 spinach leaves
- 18 vegan spring roll wrappers
- 6 slices cheese , cut into 18 smaller strips
- Water
- 1 cup vegetable oil
- 6 cups cauliflower rice
- 3 cups tomato , cubed
- 3 cups cucumber , cubed
- 1 tablespoon olive oil
- 1 teaspoon balsamic vinegar

d:

1. Place one spinach leaf on top of each wrapper.
2. Add a small strip of vegan cheese on top of each spinach leaf.
3. Roll the wrapper and seal the edges with water.
4. In a pan over medium high heat , add the vegetable oil.
5. Cook the rolls until golden brown.
6. Drain in paper towels.
7. Divide cauliflower rice into 6 food containers.
8. Add 3 cheesy spinach rolls in each food container.
9. Toss cucumber and tomato in olive oil and vinegar.
10. Place the cucumber tomato relish beside the rolls.
11. Seal and reheat in the microwave when ready to serve.

ional Value:

- *Calories 746*
- *Total Fat 38.5g*
- *Saturated Fat 10.1g*
- *Cholesterol 33mg*
- *Sodium 557mg*
- *Total Carbohydrate 86.2g*
- *Dietary Fiber 3.8g*
- *Total Sugars 2.6g*
- *Protein 18g*
- *Potassium 364mg*

illed Summer Veggies

Preparation Time: 15 minutes
King Time: 6 minutes
vings: 6

redients:

- 2 teaspoons cider vinegar
- 1 tablespoon olive oil
- ¼ teaspoon fresh thyme , chopped
- 1 teaspoon fresh parsley , chopped
- ¼ teaspoon fresh rosemary , chopped
- Salt and pepper to taste
- 1 onion , sliced into wedges
- 2 red bell peppers , sliced
- 3 tomatoes , sliced in half
- 6 large mushrooms , stems removed
- 1 eggplant , sliced crosswise
- 3 tablespoons olive oil
- 1 tablespoon cider vinegar

hod:

1. Make the dressing by mixing the vinegar , oil , thyme , parsley , rosemary , and pepper.
2. In a bowl , mix the onion , red bell pepper , tomatoes , mushrooms and egg
3. Toss in remaining olive oil and cider vinegar.
4. Grill over medium heat for 3 minutes.
5. Turn the vegetables and grill for another 3 minutes.
6. Arrange grilled vegetables in a food container.
7. Drizzle with the herbed mixture when ready to serve.

ritional Value:

- *Calories 127*
- *Total Fat 9 g*
- *Saturated Fat 1 g*
- *Cholesterol 0 mg*
- *Sodium 55 mg*
- *Total Carbohydrate 11 g*
- *Dietary Fiber 5 g*
- *Total Sugars 5 g*
- *Protein 3 g*
- *Potassium 464 mg*

erfood Buddha Bowl

ration Time: 10 minutes

ng Time: 10 minutes

igs: 4

dients:

- 8 oz. microwavable quinoa
- 2 tablespoons lemon juice
- ½ cup hummus
- Water
- 5 oz. baby kale
- 8 oz. cooked baby beets , sliced
- 1 cup frozen shelled edamame (thawed)
- ¼ cup sunflower seeds , toasted
- 1 avocado , sliced
- 1 cup pecans
- 2 tablespoons flaxseeds

d:

1. Cook quinoa according to directions in the packaging.
2. Set aside and let cool.
3. In a bowl , mix the lemon juice and hummus.
4. Add water to achieve desired consistency.
5. Divide mixture into 4 condiment containers.
6. Cover containers with lids and put in the refrigerator.
7. Divide the baby kale into 4 food containers with lids.
8. Top with quinoa , beets , edamame and sunflower seeds.
9. Store in the refrigerator until ready to serve.
10. Before serving add avocado slices and hummus dressing.

ional Value:

- *Calories 381*
- *Total Fat 19 g*
- *Saturated Fat 2 g*
- *Cholesterol 0 mg*
- *Sodium 188 mg*
- *Total Carbohydrate 43 g*
- *Dietary Fiber 13 g*
- *Total Sugars 8 g*
- *Protein 16 g*
- *Potassium 1 ,066 mg*

rrito & Cauliflower Rice Bowl

paration Time: 15 minutes

king Time: 10 minutes

ings: 4

edients:

- 1 cup cooked tofu cubes
- 12 oz. frozen cauliflower rice
- 4 teaspoons olive oil
- 1 teaspoon unsalted taco seasoning
- 1 cup red cabbage , sliced thinly
- ½ cup salsa
- ¼ cup fresh cilantro , chopped
- 1 cup avocado , diced

hod:

1. Prepare cauliflower rice according to directions in the package.
2. Toss cauliflower rice in olive oil and taco seasoning.
3. Divide among 4 food containers with lid.
4. Top with tofu , cabbage , salsa and cilantro.
5. Seal the container and chill in the refrigerator until ready to serve.
6. Before serving , add avocado slices.

ritional Value:

- *Calories 298*
- *Total Fat 20 g*
- *Saturated Fat 3 g*
- *Cholesterol 0 mg*
- *Sodium 680 mg*
- *Total Carbohydrate 15 g*
- *Dietary Fiber 6 g*
- *Total Sugars 5 g*
- *Protein 15 g*
- *Potassium 241 mg*

on Garlic Broccoli

ration Time: 10 minutes

ng Time: 10 minutes

gs: 2

dients:

- 2 teaspoons olive oil
- 3 cloves garlic , minced
- 2 cups broccoli , sliced into florets
- Salt and pepper to taste
- 1 tablespoon freshly squeezed lemon juice

d:

1. In a pan over medium heat , pour the olive oil.
2. Once hot , add the garlic and cook for 30 seconds.
3. Add the broccoli florets and cook until tender
4. Stir in the lemon juice. Let cool.
5. Put in a food container and reheat when ready to eat.

ional Value:

- *Calories 80*
- *Total Fat 5.1g*
- *Saturated Fat 0.7g*
- *Cholesterol 0mg*
- *Sodium 32mg*
- *Total Carbohydrate 7.7g*
- *Dietary Fiber 2.5g*
- *Total Sugars 1.8g*
- *Protein 2.9g*
- *Potassium 316mg*

eamed Cabbage & Carrots

paration Time: 10 minutes
king Time: 20 minutes
vings: 8
redients:

- 2 teaspoons olive oil
- 1 cup carrots , sliced
- 1 green bell pepper , sliced into strips
- 1 head green cabbage , sliced
- 2 tablespoons water
- Salt and pepper to taste

thod:

1. Pour oil in a pot over medium heat.
2. Add carrot strips and cook for 5 minutes.
3. Add bell pepper and cabbage.
4. Pour in the water and season with salt and pepper.
5. Cover the pot.
6. Cook for 15 minutes or until tender.
7. Store in food container and reheat when ready to eat.

tritional Value:

- *Calories 36*
- *Total Fat 1 g*
- *Saturated Fat 0 g*
- *Cholesterol 0 mg*
- *Sodium 168 mg*
- *Total Carbohydrate 6 g*
- *Dietary Fiber 2 g*
- *Total Sugars 3 g*
- *Protein 1 g*
- *Potassium 226 mg*

lard Greens with Shiitake Mushrooms

aration Time: 15 minutes

ng Time: 10 minutes

ıgs: 4

dients:

- ¼ teaspoon salt
- ¾ teaspoon smoked paprika
- ¼ teaspoon red pepper , crushed
- ¼ teaspoon ground cumin
- ¾ cup reduced-sodium vegetable broth
- 2 tablespoons olive oil
- 4 cloves garlic , minced
- 5 oz. shiitake mushrooms , chopped
- 16 oz. collard greens , chopped
- 2 tablespoons cider vinegar
- 1 teaspoon hot sauce
- ½ teaspoon ground pepper

d:

1. Add salt , paprika , red pepper , cumin and broth in a pan over medium heat.
2. Simmer for 1 minute , stirring to blend well.
3. Transfer to a plate and set aside.
4. In a pot over medium high heat , add the oil.
5. Cook the garlic and mushrooms for 4 minutes.
6. Pour 2 tablespoons of the paprika mixture to the pot.
7. Mix well.
8. Add the collard greens and gradually add the remaining paprika mixture.
9. Stir in the rest of the ingredients.
10. Cook for 1 minute.
11. Store in a food container and reheat when ready to eat.

onal Value:

- *Calories 120*
- *Total Fat 8 g*
- *Saturated Fat 1 g*
- *Cholesterol 0 mg*
- *Sodium 227 mg*
- *Total Carbohydrate 11 g*
- *Dietary Fiber 6 g*
- *Total Sugars 2 g*
- *Protein 5 g*
- *Potassium 384 mg*

rlic Pea Shoots

paration Time: 5 minutes
king Time: 5 minutes
ings: 6

redients:

- 2 tablespoons canola oil
- 2 tablespoons sesame oil
- 3 tablespoons garlic , minced
- 1 lb. pea shoots
- ¼ cup rice wine
- Salt and pepper to taste

hod:

1. Heat both of the oils in a pot over medium high heat.
2. Add garlic and cook for 30 seconds , stirring frequently.
3. Add pea shoots and rice wine.
4. Season with salt and pepper.
5. Cook for 3 minutes.
6. Place in a food container and heat in the microwave when ready to eat.

ritional Value:

- *Calories 150*
- *Total Fat 10 g*
- *Saturated Fat 1 g*
- *Cholesterol 0 mg*
- *Sodium 291 mg*
- *Total Carbohydrate 7 g*
- *Dietary Fiber 2 g*
- *Total Sugars 3 g*
- *Protein 2 g*
- *Potassium 3 mg*

shed Potato with Carrots & Corn

ration Time: 15 minutes

ng Time: 30 minutes

gs: 4

dients:

- Water
- 8 potatoes , peeled and cubed
- Salt
- 4 tablespoons vegan butter , divided
- 1 cup frozen corn and carrot cubes
- Salt and pepper to taste
- 1 cup pecans
- 2 tablespoons flaxseeds

d:

1. Fill a pot with water.
2. Put in the stove and bring to a boil.
3. Add the potatoes.
4. Simmer until the potatoes are tender.
5. Take the potatoes out of the pot and drain.
6. Mash the potatoes using a fork or a masher.
7. Stir in 3 tablespoons butter.
8. Season with salt and pepper.
9. In a pan over medium heat , add remaining butter.
10. Add the frozen vegetables.
11. Sauté for 3 minutes.
12. Drain the liquid.
13. Divide the mashed potato in food containers.
14. Top with the cubed corn and carrots.
15. Reheat before serving.

onal Value:

- *Calories 556*
- *Total Fat 26.5g*
- *Saturated Fat 2.8g*
- *Cholesterol 0mg*
- *Sodium 65mg*
- *Total Carbohydrate 72.9g*
- *Dietary Fiber 14.9g*
- *Total Sugars 6.2g*
- *Protein 11.6g*
- *Potassium 1908mg*

utéed Green Beans , Mushrooms & Tomatoes

paration Time: 15 minutes
king Time: 15 minutes
vings: 10
redients:

- Water
- 3 lb. green beans , trimmed
- 2 tablespoons olive oil
- 8 cloves garlic , minced
- ½ cup tomato , diced
- 12 oz. cremini mushrooms , sliced into quarters
- Salt and pepper to taste

hod:

1. Fill a pot with water.
2. Bring to a boil.
3. Add the beans and cook for 5 minutes.
4. Drain the beans.
5. Dry the pot.
6. Pour oil into the pot.
7. Add garlic , tomato and mushrooms.
8. Cook for 5 minutes.
9. Add the beans and cook for another 5 minutes.
10. Season with salt and pepper.
11. Store in a food container and reheat before eating.

ritional Value:

- *Calories 74*
- *Total Fat 3 g*
- *Saturated Fat 0 g*
- *Cholesterol 0 mg*
- *Sodium 185 mg*
- *Total Carbohydrate 11 g*
- *Dietary Fiber 4 g*
- *Total Sugars 5 g*
- *Protein 3 g*
- *Potassium 438 mg*

on Mustard Baby Veggies

ration Time: 15 minutes

ng Time: 10 minutes

gs: 8

dients:

- 1 clove garlic , minced
- 2 tablespoons fresh lemon juice
- 1 teaspoon Dijon mustard
- 2 tablespoons olive oil , divided
- 2 tablespoons water
- ½ teaspoon lemon zest
- 2 teaspoons fresh basil , chopped
- 1 lb. baby zucchini
- ½ lb. baby carrots
- ½ lb. baby potatoes
- 12 cherry tomatoes

d:

1. Mix garlic , lemon juice , mustard , half of olive oil , water and lemon zest in a bowl.
2. Transfer to a glass jar with lid.
3. Pour remaining olive oil in a pan over medium heat.
4. Once hot , add the vegetables.
5. Cook until tender.
6. Drain and transfer in a food container.
7. When ready to eat , reheat veggies and toss in the lemon mustard sauce.

onal Value:

- *Calories 57*
- *Total Fat 2 g*
- *Saturated Fat 0 g*
- *Cholesterol 0 mg*
- *Sodium 190 mg*
- *Total Carbohydrate 9 g*
- *Dietary Fiber 3 g*
- *Total Sugars 5 g*
- *Protein 2 g*
- *Potassium 343 mg*

Roasted Vegetables in Balsamic Sauce

Preparation Time: 10 minutes

Cooking Time: 23 minutes

Servings: 12

Ingredients:

- 1 onion , sliced into wedges
- 2 cloves garlic , minced
- 1 lb. green beans , trimmed
- 2 tablespoons olive oil
- Salt and pepper to taste
- 4 yellow summer squash , sliced
- ⅔ cup balsamic vinegar

Method:

1. Preheat your oven to 450 degrees F.
2. Toss onion , garlic and beans in olive oil.
3. Transfer to a baking pan.
4. Season with salt and pepper.
5. Roast in the oven for 8 minutes.
6. Add the squash.
7. Roast for another 5 minutes.
8. In a pan over medium high heat , pour the balsamic vinegar and bring to a
9. Reduce heat and simmer for 10 minutes.
10. Transfer roasted vegetables in a food container.
11. Reheat the veggies and toss in balsamic vinegar sauce when ready to ser

Nutritional Value:

- *Calories 90*
- *Total Fat 4 g*
- *Saturated Fat 1 g*
- *Cholesterol 0 mg*
- *Sodium 45 mg*
- *Total Carbohydrate 13 g*
- *Dietary Fiber 3 g*
- *Total Sugars 9 g*
- *Protein 2 g*
- *Potassium 45 mg*

sted Root Vegetables

rration Time: 20 minutes

ng Time: 1 hour and 10 minutes

gs: 8

dients:

- 2 cups celery root , sliced
- 1 ½ cups baby carrots , peeled
- 8 oz. baby potatoes , sliced in half
- 3 parsnips , sliced
- 1 fennel bulb , cored and quartered
- 2 shallots , sliced
- 2 tablespoons olive oil
- Salt and pepper to taste

d:

1. Preheat your oven to 325 degrees F.
2. In a baking pan , put all the root vegetables and toss to combine.
3. Drizzle with oil and season with salt and pepper.
4. Mix well.
5. Bake for 1 hour.
6. Increase temperature of your oven to 425 degrees F.
7. Bake for 10 minutes.
8. Transfer to a food container.
9. Reheat in pan without oil before serving.

ional Value:

- *Calories 82*
- *Total Fat 2 g*
- *Saturated Fat 0 g*
- *Cholesterol 0 mg*
- *Sodium 136 mg*
- *Total Carbohydrate 14 g*
- *Dietary Fiber 3 g*
- *Total Sugars 4 g*
- *Protein 2 g*
- *Potassium 407 mg*

een Beans , Roasted Red Peppers & Onions

paration Time: 15 minutes

king Time: 25 minutes

ings: 6

redients:

- 1 tablespoon olive oil
- 1 ½ cups onion , chopped
- 1 tablespoon red wine vinegar
- ½ cup jarred roasted red peppers , drained and chopped
- 2 tablespoons fresh basil , chopped
- ¼ cup olives , pitted and sliced
- Salt and pepper to taste
- 1 lb. fresh green beans , trimmed and sliced

hod:

1. Pour olive oil in a pan over medium heat.
2. Add onion and cook for 10 minutes.
3. Pour in the vinegar.
4. Cook for 2 minutes.
5. Add roasted red peppers , basil and olives.
6. Season with salt and pepper.
7. Remove from the stove.
8. In a saucepan with water , cook beans for 10 minutes.
9. Add beans to the onion mixture.
10. Stir for 3 minutes.

ritional Value:

- *Calories 73*
- *Total Fat 3 g*
- *Saturated Fat 0 g*
- *Cholesterol 0 mg*
- *Sodium 153 mg*
- *Total Carbohydrate 11 g*
- *Dietary Fiber 4 g*
- *Total Sugars 3 g*
- *Protein 2 g*
- *Potassium 248 mg*

ccoli & Cauliflower in Lemon-Dill Sauce

ration Time: 10 minutes

ng Time: 20 minutes

1gs: 4

dients:

- 1 tablespoon olive oil
- 2 teaspoons lemon juice
- ½ teaspoon dried dill weed
- 1 clove garlic , minced
- Salt and pepper to taste
- ⅛ teaspoon dry mustard
- 2 cups cauliflower florets
- 2 cups broccoli florets
- Fresh dill sprigs

d:

1. Preheat your oven to 375 degrees F.
2. Add olive oil , lemon juice , dill , garlic , salt , pepper and mustard in a glass ja with lid.
3. Shake to blend well.
4. In a baking pan , toss cauliflower and broccoli in 3 tablespoons lemon dill sa
5. Bake in the oven for 20 minutes or until tender.
6. Toss in the remaining sauce before serving.

ional Value:

- *Calories 60*
- *Total Fat 4 g*
- *Saturated Fat 1 g*
- *Cholesterol 0 mg*
- *Sodium 103 mg*
- *Total Carbohydrate 6 g*
- *Dietary Fiber 2 g*
- *Total Sugars 2 g*
- *Protein 2 g*
- *Potassium 301 mg*

getable Salad in Mason Jar

paration Time: 5 minutes

king Time: 0 minute

vings: 1

redients:

- 2 tablespoons cashew sauce (recipe in the sauce section)
- 1 cup tofu cubes , roasted
- 1 tablespoon pumpkin seeds
- 1 cup carrots , roasted
- 2 cups mixed greens

hod:

1. In a glass jar , layer the cashew sauce , tofu , seeds , carrots and mixed gree
2. Seal the jar.
3. Refrigerate up to 5 days.
4. Serve whenever ready to eat.

ritional Value:

- *Calories 400*
- *Total Fat 27 g*
- *Saturated Fat 5 g*
- *Cholesterol 0 mg*
- *Sodium 383 mg*
- *Total Carbohydrate 21 g*
- *Dietary Fiber 8 g*
- *Total Sugars 5 g*
- *Protein 27 g*
- *Potassium 895 mg*

et Spicy Beans

ration Time: 10 minutes

ng Time: 50 minutes

gs: 10

dients:

- 3 tablespoons vegetable oil
- 1 onion , chopped
- 45 oz. navy beans , rinsed and drained
- 1 ½ cups water
- ¾ cup ketchup
- ⅓ cup brown sugar
- 1 tablespoon white vinegar
- 1 teaspoon chipotle peppers in adobo sauce
- Salt and pepper to taste

d:

1. Pour the oil in a pan over medium heat.
2. Add onion and cook for 10 minutes.
3. Add the rest of the ingredients.
4. Bring to a boil.
5. Reduce heat and simmer for 30 minutes.
6. Transfer to food container.
7. Reheat when ready to eat.

onal Value:

- *Calories 191*
- *Total Fat 4 g*
- *Saturated Fat 0 g*
- *Cholesterol 0 mg*
- *Sodium 354 mg*
- *Total Carbohydrate 32 g*
- *Dietary Fiber 7 g*
- *Total Sugars 12 g*
- *Protein 7 g*
- *Potassium 361 mg*

amame & Aleppo Pepper

paration Time: 5 minutes

king Time: 5 minutes

ving: 1

redients:

- ½ cup edamame pods
- Water
- ⅛ teaspoon Aleppo pepper

thod:

1. Place edamame pods in a steamer basket.
2. Put the basket on top of a pot with water.
3. Steam.
4. Store in glass jar with lid.
5. Season with Aleppo pepper before serving.

ritional Value:

- *Calories 101*
- *Total Fat 3 g*
- *Saturated Fat 0 g*
- *Cholesterol 0 mg*
- *Sodium 30 mg*
- *Total Carbohydrate 9 g*
- *Dietary Fiber 4 g*
- *Total Sugars 1 g*
- *Protein 8 g*
- *Potassium 4 mg*

hi Grain Meal

ration Time: 20 minutes

ng Time: 0 minute

ıgs: 4

dients:

- 2 teaspoons fresh ginger , grated
- 2 tablespoons low sodium tamari
- 2 tablespoons rice vinegar
- 2 teaspoons sesame oil , toasted
- 2 tablespoons avocado oil
- 2 cups brown rice , cooked
- 1 cup cucumber , diced
- 1 cup carrot , shredded
- 1 avocado , diced
- 1 cup toasted nori , chopped
- 1 cup shelled edamame , cooked
- Sesame seeds

d:

1. In a bowl , mix the ginger , tamari , vinegar , sesame oil and avocado oil.
2. Divide brown rice among 4 food containers with lids.
3. Top with the cucumber , carrot , avocado , nori and edamame.
4. Sprinkle sesame seeds on top.
5. Seal the container and refrigerate.
6. Drizzle sauce on top when ready to eat.

ional Value:

- *Calories 341*
- *Total Fat 20 g*
- *Saturated Fat 3 g*
- *Cholesterol 0 mg*
- *Sodium 381 mg*
- *Total Carbohydrate 35 g*
- *Dietary Fiber 8 g*
- *Total Sugars 3 g*
- *Protein 20 g*
- *Potassium 596 mg*

inoa & Snap Pea Salad

paration Time: 20 minutes

king Time: 20 minutes

ings: 6

redients:

- 2 cups water
- 1 cup quinoa
- ⅓ cup onion , sliced
- 1 ½ cups mushrooms , sliced
- 1 tablespoon fresh dill , chopped
- 2 cups fresh snap peas , trimmed and sliced
- ⅓ cup white wine vinegar
- ¼ cup flaxseed oil
- 1 teaspoon lemon zest
- 1 tablespoon lemon juice
- 1 teaspoon maple syrup

hod:

1. Put quinoa and water in a pan over medium high heat.
2. Bring to a boil.
3. Reduce heat and simmer for 15 minutes.
4. Fluff using a fork and set aside.
5. In a bowl , combine onion , mushrooms , dill and peas.
6. In another bowl , mix the rest of the ingredients.
7. Transfer the quinoa in a food container.
8. Stir in the pea mixture.
9. Seal the container and refrigerate until ready to serve.
10. Transfer the maple dressing into a glass jar with lid.
11. Drizzle dressing over the quinoa salad before serving.

ritional Value:

- *Calories 223*
- *Total Fat 11 g*
- *Saturated Fat 2 g*
- *Cholesterol 0 mg*
- *Sodium 10 mg*
- *Total Carbohydrate 25 g*
- *Dietary Fiber 3 g*
- *Total Sugars 6 g*
- *Protein 6 g*
- *Potassium 311 mg*

ckpea & Quinoa

ration Time: 15 minutes

ng Time: 0 minute

1g: 1

dients:

- 3 tablespoons hummus
- 1 tablespoon lemon juice
- 1 tablespoon roasted red pepper , chopped
- 1 tablespoon water
- Salt and pepper to taste
- 1 cup cooked quinoa
- ¼ avocado , diced
- ⅓ cup canned chickpeas , rinsed and drained
- ½ cup cherry tomatoes , sliced in half
- ½ cup cucumber , sliced

d:

1. In a glass jar with lid , mix the hummus , lemon juice , red pepper , water , sal and pepper.
2. Shake to mix.
3. Arrange the rest of the ingredients in a food container.
4. Drizzle with sauce when ready to eat.

ional Value:

- *Calories 503*
- *Total Fat 17 g*
- *Saturated Fat 2 g*
- *Cholesterol 0 mg*
- *Sodium 573 mg*
- *Total Carbohydrate 75 g*
- *Dietary Fiber 16 g*
- *Total Sugars 6 g*
- *Protein 18 g*
- *Potassium 1 ,083 mg*

ets , Edamame & Mixed Green Salad

Preparation Time: 10 minutes

Cooking Time: 0 minute

Serving: 1

Ingredients:

- 2 cups mixed greens
- ½ raw beet , peeled and shredded
- 1 cup shelled edamame , thawed
- 1 tablespoon red wine vinegar
- 1 tablespoon fresh cilantro , chopped
- 2 teaspoons extra-virgin olive oil
- Pepper to taste

Method:

1. Place the mixed greens in a food container.
2. Top with shredded beets and edamame.
3. In a glass jar with lid , mix the rest of the ingredients.
4. Refrigerate the salad and drizzle with the dressing when ready to eat.

Nutritional Value:

- *Calories 325*
- *Total Fat 16 g*
- *Saturated Fat 1 g*
- *Cholesterol 0 mg*
- *Sodium 682 mg*
- *Total Carbohydrate 25 g*
- *Dietary Fiber 12 g*
- *Total Sugars 6 g*
- *Protein 18 g*
- *Potassium 499 mg*

ck Bean & Corn Salad

ration Time: 15 minutes

ng Time: 0 minute

gs: 4

dients:

- 2 tablespoons olive oil
- ¼ cup lime juice
- ¼ cup fresh cilantro , chopped
- Salt and pepper to taste
- 2 cups red cabbage , shredded
- 2 ¼ cups corn kernels
- ⅓ cup pine nuts , toasted
- 30 oz. canned black beans , rinsed and drained
- 1 tomato , diced
- ½ cup red onion , minced

d:

1. In a glass jar with lid , blend the oil , lime juice , cilantro , salt and pepper.
2. In a food container , arrange the red cabbage , topped with the rest of the ingredients.
3. Cover and refrigerate until ready to serve.
4. Drizzle with dressing before serving.

onal Value:

- *Calories 415*
- *Total Fat 16 g*
- *Saturated Fat 2 g*
- *Cholesterol 0 mg*
- *Sodium 480 mg*
- *Total Carbohydrate 58 g*
- *Dietary Fiber 14 g*
- *Total Sugars 16 g*
- *Protein 16 g*
- *Potassium 1 ,112 mg*

ack Beans with Rice

paration Time: 20 minutes
king Time: 2 hours and 15 minutes
vings: 8

redients:

- 1 lb. dried black beans , soaked in water overnight , rinsed and drained
- 8 cups water , divided
- 2 tablespoons dried oregano
- 1 bay leaf
- 6 cloves garlic , crushed
- 2 teaspoons olive oil
- 1 onion , chopped
- 1 red bell pepper , chopped
- 1 tablespoon ground cumin
- 1 jalapeño pepper , chopped
- 2 tablespoons balsamic vinegar
- Salt and pepper to taste
- 2 cups long-grain white rice
- 8 lime wedges

thod:

1. Put black beans in a pot.
2. Add 4 cups water , oregano , bay leaf and garlic.
3. Bring to a boil.
4. Reduce heat and simmer for 2 hours.
5. Drain and put beans back to the pot.
6. Pour in the oil.
7. Add onion and bell pepper. Cook for 5 minutes.
8. Add jalapeño pepper and cumin. Cook for 1 minute.
9. Season with salt and pepper.
10. In another saucepan , add remaining water and salt.
11. Add rice and cover.
12. Bring to a boil and then simmer for 15 minutes.
13. Put rice in a food container and top with beans.
14. Garnish with lemon wedges.
15. Refrigerate and then reheat before serving.

ritional Value:

- *Calories 600*
- *Total Fat 2 g*
- *Saturated Fat 0 g*
- *Cholesterol 0 mg*
- *Sodium 407 mg*
- *Total Carbohydrate 117 g*
- *Dietary Fiber 11 g*
- *Total Sugars 7 g*

- *Protein 24 g*
- *Potassium 230 mg*

ow Cooked Beans

paration Time: 10 minutes

king Time: 2 hours and 15 minutes

vings: 4

redients:

- 1 lb. black beans , soaked overnight , rinsed and drained
- 1 onion , chopped
- 1 bay leaf
- 4 cloves garlic , minced
- 1 teaspoon dried thyme
- 5 cups boiling water
- Salt to taste

hod:

1. Add the beans to a slow cooker.
2. Stir in onion , bay leaf , garlic and thyme.
3. Add water and cover the pot.
4. Cook for 2 hours.
5. Season with salt and cook for another 15 minutes.

ritional Value:

- *Calories 253*
- *Total Fat 1 g*
- *Saturated Fat 0 g*
- *Cholesterol 0 mg*
- *Sodium 201 mg*
- *Total Carbohydrate 48 g*
- *Dietary Fiber 19 g*
- *Total Sugars 1 g*
- *Protein 15 g*
- *Potassium 712 mg*

...go with Quinoa & Black Beans

...ration Time: 30 minutes

...ng Time: 30 minutes

...gs: 2

...dients:

- ½ cup quinoa , toasted
- 1 cup water
- ¼ cup orange juice
- ¼ cup fresh cilantro , chopped
- 2 tablespoons rice vinegar
- 2 teaspoons sesame oil , toasted
- 1 teaspoon fresh ginger , minced
- Salt to taste
- Cayenne pepper to taste
- 1 mango , diced
- 1 red bell pepper , diced
- 1 cup canned black beans
- 2 scallions , sliced thinly

...d:

1. Put quinoa in a pot.
2. Pour in water.
3. Bring to a boil.
4. Reduce heat to simmer for 20 minutes.
5. While waiting , mix the rest of the ingredients.
6. Add the quinoa to the mango mixture and transfer to a food container.
7. Refrigerate for up to 2 days.
8. Serve chilled.

...onal Value:

- *Calories 419*
- *Total Fat 9 g*
- *Saturated Fat 1 g*
- *Cholesterol 0 mg*
- *Sodium 256 mg*
- *Total Carbohydrate 72 g*
- *Dietary Fiber 20 g*
- *Total Sugars 25 g*
- *Protein 15 g*
- *Potassium 964 mg*

mato Salsa with Marjoram

paration Time: 10 minutes

king Time: 0 minute

ings: 12

redients:

- 1 clove garlic , minced
- ½ teaspoon salt
- 3 tomatoes , chopped
- 2 tablespoons white onion , chopped
- 2 teaspoons fresh marjoram , chopped
- Pepper to taste

hod:

1. Mash garlic using a fork.
2. Season with salt.
3. Mix the rest of the ingredients with the garlic paste.
4. Use as dip for vegan chips and crackers.

ritional Value:

- *Calories 5*
- *Total Fat 0 g*
- *Saturated Fat 0 g*
- *Cholesterol 0 mg*
- *Sodium 81 mg*
- *Total Carbohydrate 1 g*
- *Dietary Fiber 0 g*
- *Total Sugars 1 g*
- *Protein 0 g*
- *Potassium 58 mg*

on Garlic Tahini Sauce

ration Time: 10 minutes

ng Time: 0 minute

gs: 8

dients:

- 3 tablespoons tahini
- 3 tablespoons warm water
- 2 tablespoons lemon juice
- 1 tablespoon olive oil
- 1 clove garlic , grated
- Salt to taste

d:

1. Combine all the ingredients in a glass jar with lid.
2. Shake to blend well.
3. Cover and refrigerate until ready to use.

ional Value:

- *Calories 50*
- *Total Fat 5 g*
- *Saturated Fat 1 g*
- *Cholesterol 0 mg*
- *Sodium 75 mg*
- *Total Carbohydrate 2 g*
- *Dietary Fiber 0 g*
- *Total Sugars 0 g*
- *Protein 1 g*
- *Potassium 35 mg*

ushroom Gravy

paration Time: 10 minutes
king Time: 10 minutes
vings: 8

redients:

- 3 tablespoons olive oil
- 1 cup button mushrooms
- 1 cup cremini mushrooms
- 1 cup oyster mushrooms
- 1 cup shiitake mushrooms
- Salt and pepper to taste
- 1 shallot , chopped
- ¼ cup dry sherry
- 2 tablespoons all-purpose flour
- 2 cups mushroom broth
- 1 teaspoon fresh thyme , chopped

thod:

1. Pour oil into a pan over medium high heat.
2. Add mushrooms and season with salt and pepper.
3. Cook for 3 minutes without stirring.
4. Stir and then cook for 3 more minutes.
5. Add shallot and cook for 1 minute.
6. Lower heat and pour in sherry.
7. Cook while stirring for 1 minute.
8. Sprinkle flour and mix to coat evenly.
9. Pour in the broth and bring to a boil.
10. Simmer until the sauce has been reduced.
11. Add thyme.
12. Store in the refrigerator.
13. Serve with mashed potatoes or cauliflower steaks.

ritional Value:

- *Calories 70*
- *Total Fat 5.4g*
- *Saturated Fat 0.8g*
- *Cholesterol 0mg*
- *Sodium 45mg*
- *Total Carbohydrate 5.2g*
- *Dietary Fiber 0.7g*
- *Total Sugars 1g*
- *Protein 1.2g*
- *Potassium 93mg*

per Vinaigrette

ration Time: 15 minutes

ng Time: 25 minutes

1gs: 6

dients:

- 1 red bell pepper , sliced in half
- 1 jalapeño pepper , sliced in half
- 2 tablespoons lime juice
- 2 tablespoons balsamic vinegar
- 2 tablespoons olive oil
- Salt to taste

od:

1. Preheat your oven to 425 degrees F.
2. Place peppers in a baking pan.
3. Roast for 25 minutes.
4. Add to a food processor and pulse until smooth.
5. Stir in the rest of the ingredients.
6. Use as dressing for salads.

ional Value:

- *Calories 54*
- *Total Fat 5 g*
- *Saturated Fat 1 g*
- *Cholesterol 0 mg*
- *Sodium 50 mg*
- *Total Carbohydrate 3 g*
- *Dietary Fiber 1 g*
- *Total Sugars 2 g*
- *Protein 0 g*
- *Potassium 56 mg*

eek Salad Dressing

Preparation Time: 5 minutes

king Time: 0 minute

vings: 7

redients:

- 3 tablespoons olive oil
- 1 tablespoon lemon juice
- 1 tablespoon red wine vinegar
- 1 teaspoon dried oregano
- Salt and pepper to taste

hod:

1. Mix all the ingredients in a glass jar with lid.
2. Refrigerate for up to 1 week until ready to use.

ritional Value:

- *Calories 55*
- *Total Fat 6 g*
- *Saturated Fat 1 g*
- *Cholesterol 0 mg*
- *Sodium 83 mg*
- *Total Carbohydrate 0 g*
- *Dietary Fiber 0 g*
- *Total Sugars 0 g*
- *Protein 0 g*
- *Potassium 6 mg*

...us Vinaigrette

Preparation Time: 5 minutes

Cooking Time: 0 minute

Servings: 12

Ingredients:

- 1 orange
- 2 limes
- 2 tablespoons Dijon mustard
- 4 cloves garlic , peeled
- Salt to taste
- ¼ cup olive oil

Method:

1. Squeeze juice from the orange and limes.
2. Add the fruits and their juices to the blender.
3. Add the other ingredients.
4. Blend until smooth.
5. Serve with salad or steamed veggies.

Nutritional Value:

- *Calories 45*
- *Total Fat 5 g*
- *Saturated Fat 1 g*
- *Cholesterol 0 mg*
- *Sodium 106 mg*
- *Total Carbohydrate 1 g*
- *Dietary Fiber 0 g*
- *Total Sugars 1 g*
- *Protein 0 g*
- *Potassium 21 mg*

eamy Cashew Sauce

paration Time: 5 minutes

king Time: 0 minute

ings: 8

redients:

- ¾ cup raw cashews
- ½ cup water
- ¼ cup parsley leaves
- 1 tablespoon cider vinegar
- 1 tablespoon olive oil
- ½ teaspoon low sodium tamari
- Salt to taste

hod:

1. Put all the ingredients in a blender.
2. Puree until smooth.
3. Refrigerate for up to 4 days until ready to use.

ritional Value:

- *Calories 76*
- *Total Fat 6 g*
- *Saturated Fat 1 g*
- *Cholesterol 0 mg*
- *Sodium 90 mg*
- *Total Carbohydrate 3 g*
- *Dietary Fiber 0 g*
- *Total Sugars 1 g*
- *Protein 2 g*
- *Potassium 83 mg*

co Peanut Butter

ration Time: 5 minutes

ng Time: 10 minutes

gs: 8

dients:

- 1 ¼ cups unsalted peanuts
- ⅓ cup chopped dark chocolate chips , melted
- 2 tablespoons pure maple syrup
- 1 tablespoon peanut oil
- ½ teaspoon vanilla extract
- ¼ teaspoon salt

d:

1. Preheat your oven to 350 degrees F.
2. Arrange peanuts in a single layer in a baking sheet.
3. Bake for 10 minutes.
4. Transfer to a food processor and add the rest of the ingredients.
5. Blend until smooth.
6. Store up to 1 month.

ional Value:

- *Calories 201*
- *Total Fat 15 g*
- *Saturated Fat 3 g*
- *Cholesterol 0 mg*
- *Sodium 76 mg*
- *Total Carbohydrate 12 g*
- *Dietary Fiber 2 g*
- *Total Sugars 7 g*
- *Protein 6 g*
- *Potassium 195 mg*

nger Cranberry Sauce

paration Time: 5 minutes
king Time: 10 minutes
vings: 10
redients:

- ½ cup maple syrup
- ½ cup water
- 2 tablespoons lime juice
- ⅓ cup sugar
- 1 teaspoon fresh ginger , chopped
- 3 cups cranberries

thod:

1. In a saucepan over medium high heat , add the maple syrup , water , lime j and sugar.
2. Bring to a boil.
3. Stir to dissolve the sugar.
4. Reduce heat and simmer for 3 minutes.
5. Add ginger and cranberries.
6. Simmer for 5 minutes.
7. Store in a glass jar in the refrigerator for up to 3 days.
8. Bring to room temperature for half an hour before serving.

ritional Value:

- *Calories 83*
- *Total Fat 0 g*
- *Saturated Fat 0 g*
- *Cholesterol 0 mg*
- *Sodium 2 mg*
- *Total Carbohydrate 22 g*
- *Dietary Fiber 2 g*
- *Total Sugars 17 g*
- *Protein 0 g*
- *Potassium 350 mg*

le Butter

ration Time: 5 minutes

ng Time: 45 minutes

gs: 24

dients:

- 4 lb. apples , cubed
- ½ cup sugar
- 1 cup apple cider
- 1 teaspoon ground cinnamon
- ½ teaspoon salt
- ¼ teaspoon ground ginger
- ¼ teaspoon ground cloves
- ¼ teaspoon ground nutmeg
- 1 tablespoon lemon juice

d:

1. Add apples , sugar and cider in a pan over medium high heat.
2. Bring to a boil.
3. Reduce heat and simmer for 20 minutes. Stir every 5 minutes.
4. Transfer the contents of the pan to a blender.
5. Blend until smooth.
6. Put it back to the pan.
7. Add the rest of the ingredients except lemon juice.
8. Simmer for 20 minutes.
9. Remove from heat and stir in the lemon juice.
10. Refrigerate for up to 2 weeks.

ional Value:

- *Calories 51*
- *Total Fat 0 g*
- *Saturated Fat 0 g*
- *Cholesterol 0 mg*
- *Sodium 49 mg*
- *Total Carbohydrate 13 g*
- *Dietary Fiber 1 g*
- *Total Sugars 11 g*
- *Protein 0 g*
- *Potassium 62 mg*

ocado Toasts

paration Time: 5 minutes

king Time: 0 minute

vings: 5

redients:

- 5 whole grain crackers
- ¼ avocado , mashed
- 1 tablespoon black olives , sliced
- ¼ cup tomatoes , chopped

hod:

1. Arrange whole grain crackers in a food container.
2. Spread each cracker with mashed avocado.
3. Top with black olives and tomatoes.
4. Refrigerate until ready to eat.
5. Toast in the oven before serving.

ritional Value:

- *Calories 211*
- *Total Fat 13 g*
- *Saturated Fat 2 g*
- *Cholesterol 0 mg*
- *Sodium 293 mg*
- *Total Carbohydrate 23 g*
- *Dietary Fiber 6 g*
- *Total Sugars 5 g*
- *Protein 4 g*
- *Potassium 424 mg*

eet & Spicy Snack Mix

ration Time: 5 minutes

ng Time: 18 minutes

gs: 20

dients:

- 4 cups mixed vegetable sticks
- ½ cup whole almonds
- 2 cups corn square cereal
- 2 cups oat cereal , toasted
- 1 ¾ cups pretzel sticks
- 1 teaspoon packed brown sugar
- 1 teaspoon paprika
- ½ teaspoon chili powder
- ½ teaspoon ground cumin
- ¼ teaspoon cayenne pepper
- Salt to taste
- Cooking spray

d:

1. Preheat your oven to 300 degrees F.
2. In a roasting pan , add the vegetable sticks , almonds , corn and oat cereals ar pretzel sticks.
3. In a bowl , mix the rest of the ingredients.
4. Coat the cereal mixture with cooking spray.
5. Sprinkle spice mixture on top of the cereals.
6. Bake in the oven for 18 minutes.
7. Store in an airtight container for up to 7 days.

onal Value:

- *Calories 92*
- *Total Fat 3 g*
- *Saturated Fat 0 g*
- *Cholesterol 0 mg*
- *Sodium 228 mg*
- *Total Carbohydrate 13 g*
- *Dietary Fiber 1 g*
- *Total Sugars 1 g*
- *Protein 2 g*
- *Potassium 28 mg*

rrot & Peppers with Hummus

paration Time: 5 minutes

king Time: 0 minute

ying: 1

redients:

- ½ green bell pepper , sliced
- 2 carrots , sliced into sticks
- 3 tablespoons hummus

hod:

1. Arrange carrot and pepper slices in a food container.
2. Place hummus in a smaller food container and add to the big food containe beside the carrot and peppers.

ritional Value:

- *Calories 140*
- *Total Fat 5 g*
- *Saturated Fat 1 g*
- *Cholesterol 0 mg*
- *Sodium 264 mg*
- *Total Carbohydrate 21 g*
- *Dietary Fiber 7 g*
- *Total Sugars 7 g*
- *Protein 5 g*
- *Potassium 601 mg*

sted Squash Seeds

ration Time: 10 minutes

ng Time: 15 minutes

gs: 2

dients:

- ½ cup spaghetti squash seeds
- ½ teaspoon olive oil
- 1 teaspoon maple syrup
- ½ teaspoon ground cumin
- ½ teaspoon ground cinnamon
- ⅛ teaspoon salt

d:

1. Preheat your oven to 300 degrees F.
2. Toss seeds in the mixture of the rest of the ingredients.
3. Spread on a baking sheet.
4. Bake for 15 minutes.
5. Store in airtight container.

ional Value:

- *Calories 203*
- *Total Fat 17 g*
- *Saturated Fat 3 g*
- *Cholesterol 0 mg*
- *Sodium 74 mg*
- *Total Carbohydrate 6 g*
- *Dietary Fiber 2 g*
- *Total Sugars 2 g*
- *Protein 10 g*
- *Potassium 271 mg*

ips with Kiwi Salsa

paration Time: 5 minutes
king Time: 0 minute
vings: 1

redients:

- 2 tablespoons kiwi , chopped
- 2 tablespoons tomato salsa
- 8 corn tortilla chips

thod:

1. Combine the kiwi and salsa.
2. Serve with tortilla chips.

ritional Value:

- *Calories 158*
- *Total Fat 6 g*
- *Saturated Fat 1 g*
- *Cholesterol 0 mg*
- *Sodium 334 mg*
- *Total Carbohydrate 25 g*
- *Dietary Fiber 2 g*
- *Total Sugars 3 g*
- *Protein 2 g*
- *Potassium 122 mg*

on Dessert

aration Time: 5 minutes

ng Time: 0 minute

gs: 6

dients:

- 4 cups melon balls
- ½ cup sparkling water (berry flavor)
- 3 tablespoons white balsamic vinegar
- Lemon zest

d:

1. Mix sparkling water and vinegar in a bowl.
2. Toss melon balls in the mixture.
3. Transfer to a glass jar with lid.
4. Cover and refrigerate until ready to serve.
5. Garnish with lemon zest before serving.

ional Value:

- *Calories 47*
- *Total Fat 0 g*
- *Saturated Fat 0 g*
- *Cholesterol 0 mg*
- *Sodium 16 mg*
- *Total Carbohydrate 11 g*
- *Dietary Fiber 1 g*
- *Total Sugars 10 g*
- *Protein 1 g*
- *Potassium 241 mg*

Mango & Strawberry Ice Cream

Preparation Time: 10 minutes

Cooking Time: 0 minute

Servings: 4

Ingredients:

- 12 oz. mango cubes
- 8 oz. strawberry slices
- 1 tablespoon freshly squeeze lime juice

Method:

1. Put all the ingredients in a food processor.
2. Blend until smooth.
3. Store in the freezer for up to 3 months.
4. Let it soften a little for 30 minutes before serving.

Nutritional Value:

- *Calories 70*
- *Total Fat 0 g*
- *Saturated Fat 0 g*
- *Cholesterol 0 mg*
- *Sodium 1 mg*
- *Total Carbohydrate 17 g*
- *Dietary Fiber 2 g*
- *Total Sugars 14 g*
- *Protein 1 g*
- *Potassium 234 mg*

termelon Pizza

ration Time: 10 minutes

ng Time: 0 minute

1gs: 8

dients:

- ¼ teaspoon vanilla extract
- 1 teaspoon maple syrup
- ½ cup coconut-milk yogurt
- 2 large round slices watermelon from the center
- ⅔ cup strawberries , sliced
- ½ cup blackberries , sliced in half
- 2 tablespoons unsweetened coconut flakes , toasted

od:

1. Mix vanilla , maple and yogurt in a bowl.
2. Spread mixture on top of each watermelon slice.
3. Cut into 8 slices.
4. Top with blackberries and strawberries.
5. Sprinkle coconut flakes on top.

ional Value:

- *Calories 70*
- *Total Fat 2 g*
- *Saturated Fat 1 g*
- *Cholesterol 0 mg*
- *Sodium 5 mg*
- *Total Carbohydrate 15 g*
- *Dietary Fiber 1 g*
- *Total Sugars 11 g*
- *Protein 1 g*
- *Potassium 196 mg*

asted Mango & Coconut

paration Time: 5 minutes

king Time: 10 minutes

vings: 4

redients:

- 2 mangoes , cubed
- 2 tablespoons coconut flakes
- 2 teaspoons orange zest
- 2 teaspoons crystallized ginger , chopped

hod:

1. Preheat your oven to 350 degrees F.
2. Put the mango cubes in custard cups.
3. Top with coconut flakes , orange zest and ginger.
4. Bake in the oven for 10 minutes.

ritional Value:

- *Calories 89*
- *Total Fat 2 g*
- *Saturated Fat 1 g*
- *Cholesterol 0 mg*
- *Sodium 14 mg*
- *Total Carbohydrate 20 g*
- *Dietary Fiber 2 g*
- *Total Sugars 17 g*
- *Protein 1 g*
- *Potassium 177 mg*

it Compote

ration Time: 15 minutes
ng Time: 8 hours
gs: 10

dients:

- 3 pears , cubed
- 15 oz. pineapple chunks
- ¾ cup dried apricots , sliced into quarters
- 3 tablespoons orange juice concentrate
- 1 tablespoon quick-cooking tapioca
- ½ teaspoon ground ginger
- 2 cups dark sweet cherries , pitted
- ¼ cup coconut flakes , toasted

d:

1. In a slow cooker , add all the ingredients except the cherries and coconut flak
2. Cover the pot and cook on low setting for 8 hours.
3. Stir in the cherries.
4. Transfer to food containers.
5. Sprinkle with coconut flakes.
6. Refrigerate and serve when ready to eat.

ional Value:

- *Calories 124*
- *Total Fat 1 g*
- *Saturated Fat 1 g*
- *Cholesterol 0 mg*
- *Sodium 10 mg*
- *Total Carbohydrate 29 g*
- *Dietary Fiber 3 g*
- *Total Sugars 23 g*
- *Protein 1 g*
- *Potassium 275 mg*

nclusion

oming a vegan may not be an easy fear , particularly if you are a meat-lover.
if you will consider all the benefits that it can bring to your health , and at the sam
e , how this lifestyle helps animals , it would be much easier to set your mind to ma
transition.

nember , you do not have to do it drastically.
can start gradually , and then by the time you have made the switch; you will star
erience all the wonderful benefits that veganism can bring to your life.
oy!

CPSIA information can be obtained
at www.ICGtesting.com
Printed in the USA
LVHW051802250421
685458LV00014B/1140